Contents

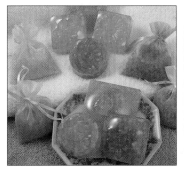
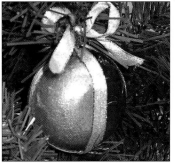
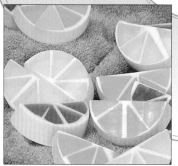
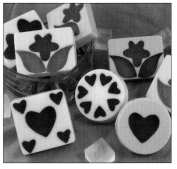
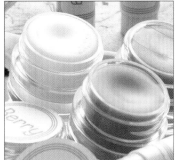
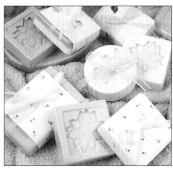
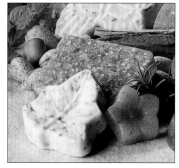
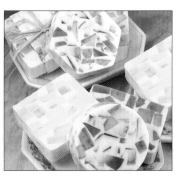
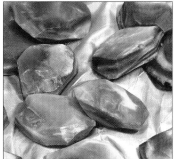
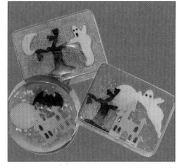
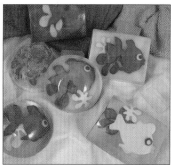
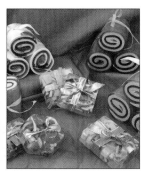
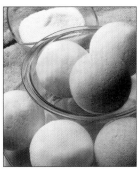
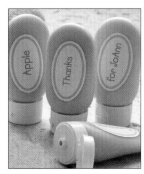
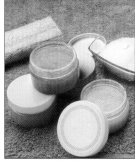
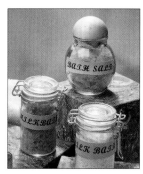

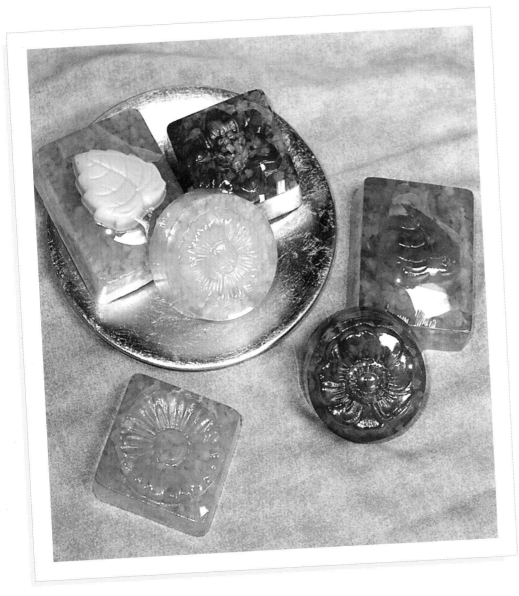

BASIC MATERIALS:
2 lb. Clear glycerin soap brick
 - *LOTP 52001*
Soap Fragrance - *LOTP*
32 oz. Bath Salts - *LOTP 61007*
Liquid Soap Colorant - *LOTP*

SUPPLIES:
Soap Kettle/Ladle - *LOTP 40000*
Sachet Bags - *LOTP 61006*
Flower Bar Mold - *LOTP 15170*
Wooden craft sticks or spoons
Two 16 oz. glass measuring cups
Kitchen knife • Small spoon • Rubbing
alcohol in a spray bottle
Plastic wrap • Scissors • Optional deco
rative paper, ribbon or raffia

Bath Salt Soap Bar

SOAP KETTLE MELTING:
1. Cut Clear soap brick into cubes with
knife and place into Soap Kettle. • 2. Me
soap in Soap Kettle, following manufacturer's instructions.

MICROWAVE MELTING:
1. Cut Clear soap brick into cubes and
place into a microwave-safe measuring
cup. • 2. Heat for 40 seconds, then in 1(
second intervals until soap is complete
melted. Stir between melting intervals.

INSTRUCTIONS:
1. Carefully ladle approximately ½ cup
melted soap in a large glass measuring cu
2. Add liquid colorant and fragrance to
melted soap. Stir until well blended.
3. Pour a small amount of soap into mo
cavities, filling slightly above the flower
portion of each mold. Spray with rubbi▶
alcohol.
4. Let poured soap set for approximate▶
5 minutes.
5. Spray mold cavities with rubbing alcoh
6. Sprinkle a small handful of salts on to
of the semi hardened soap in the mold
cavities.
7. Ladle another ½ cup of melted Clear
soap into glass measuring cup. Add fragrance and liquid colorant to melted
soap; if desired, use a different color fo▶
layered effect. Stir until well blended.
7. Pour a thin layer soap covering the
bath salts.
8. Let soap set for approximately 5 minute
10. Repeat steps 6-10, but this time pou
enough melted soap to completely fill
mold cavities.
11. Let soap set 30-40 minutes.
12. Release bars by applying constant
even pressure with thumbs on the back
side of the mold.
13. Tightly wrap soap bars in plastic wrap
14. Wrap decorative paper around finished soap bar, tie a pretty ribbon or ra
fia around bar.

Bath Salt Bars & Sachets

*Glycerin is a natural emollient
that draws moisture out of the air
to benefit skin health. It cleans
without upsetting the pH balance
necessary for soft, healthy skin.
Since LOTP uses vegetable oils,
the soap rinses clean leaving no
soapy film behind.*

*Bath salts are a great way to
add trace minerals while gently
cleansing and exfoliating the skin.*

*While waiting for soap bars to
set, make Bath Salt Sachet Bags.
Using more than one color to tint
the bath salts gives you a dramatic effect!*

*Following is a list of common
minerals found in bath salts.*

Sodium is a natural cleanser.

Magnesium is a natural skin
toner, refresher, allergy fighter and
moisture retainer.

Calcium protects against the
effects of sun damage.

Sulfate works with potassium to
preserve the alkalinity of the body's
fluid and keeps the skin healthy.

Iron is necessary for hemoglobin
formation. A deficiency of iron
results in paleness of the skin.

Silica is a natural skin toner.

Sulfur is often called "Nature's
Beauty Mineral" because it keeps the
complexion clear and youthful.

Bath Salt Sachet Bags

MATERIALS:

1 cup of Epsom salt
1 cup of sea or rock salt
    or 32 oz. Bath Salts - *LOTP 61007*
Food coloring
    or Liquid Soap Colorant - *LOTP*
20 drops of Soap Fragrance - *LOTP*

INSTRUCTIONS:

1. Empty bath salts into a glass measuring cup.
2. Add fragrance, a couple drops at a time, mixing after each addition, until desired fragrance intensity has been reached.
3. Add liquid colorant, a few drops at a time, mixing after each addition, until desired color has been reached.
4. Measure about 2 tablespoons of bath salts into each sachet bag or empty into airtight decorative container for future use.

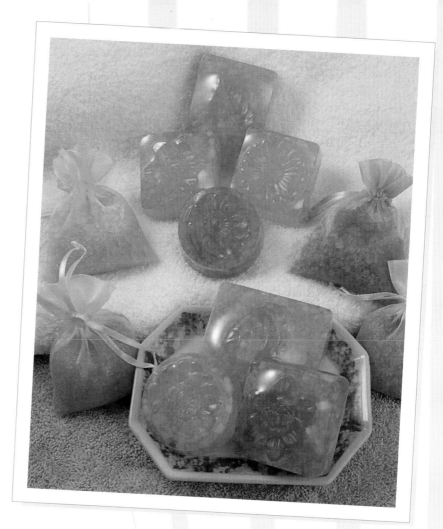

Basic Soap Bar Recipe

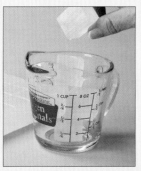 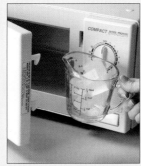 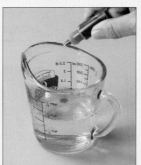 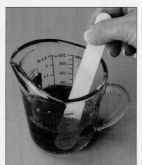 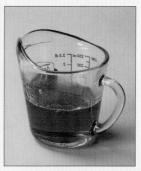

Cut soap in 1" chunks, place in microwave bowl or measuring cup. • Heat in microwave for 40 seconds, then in 10 second intervals until melted. Stir between melting intervals. • Add a very small amount of color and fragrance. • Stir melted soap slowly with a craft stick or spoon.

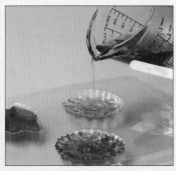 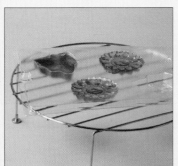 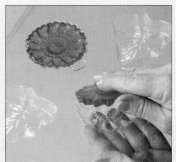 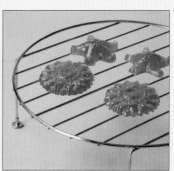

Pour slowly into mold. • Cool from 10 to 30 minutes until hard. • Pop out of mold. For easy removal, place in refrigerator for a few minutes.

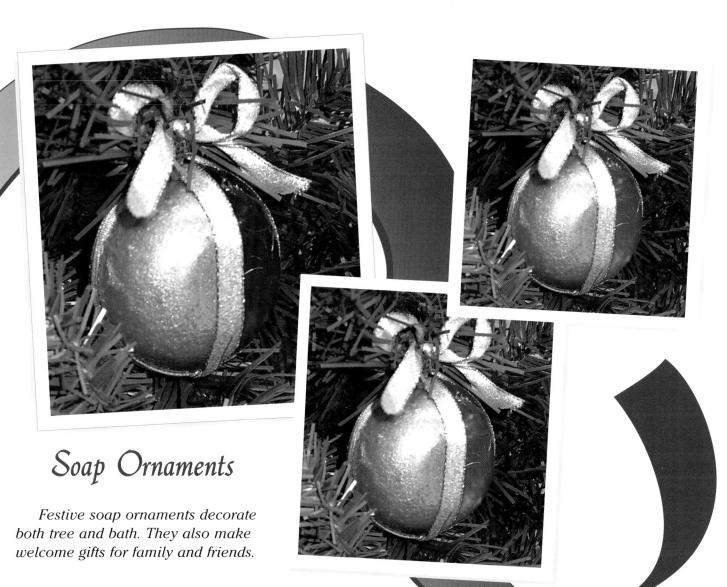

Soap Ornaments

Festive soap ornaments decorate both tree and bath. They also make welcome gifts for family and friends.

MATERIALS:
2 lbs. Clear Glycerin Soap Brick - *LOTP 52001*
Gold Colorizing Powder - *LOTP 59004*
Red or Green or Blue Soap Dye - *LOTP 53001*
Vanilla Soap Fragrance - *LOTP 51005*

SUPPLIES:
Soap Kettle/Ladle - *LOTP 40000*
Tip: A microwave oven can be used instead of the soap kettle.
Oval Round Mold - *LOTP 15152*
Microwave-safe measuring cup
⅜" wide ribbon
Kitchen knife
Spoon or craft stick
Rubbing alcohol in a spray bottle
Cutting board
Plastic wrap
Scissors

SOAP KETTLE MELTING INSTRUCTIONS:
1. Cut Clear soap brick into cubes with knife and place into Soap Kettle.
2. Melt soap in Soap Kettle, following manufacturer's instructions.

MICROWAVE MELTING INSTRUCTIONS:
1. Cut Clear soap brick into cubes and place into a microwave-safe measuring cup.
2. Heat for 40 seconds, then in 10-second intervals until soap is completely melted. Stir between melting intervals.

ORNAMENT PREPARATION:
1. You will need approximately ½ cup of melted soap to fill one of the round soap bar cavities of the soap mold. Prop the mold so that it doesn't tip when you pour the melted soap into it.
2. Red soap: Add a few drops of fragrance and Red liquid colorant to melted soap. Stir until well blended.
3. Pour into the mold, filling 1 of the cavities completely. Spray lightly with rubbing alcohol to remove air bubbles.
4. Let soap completely cool. Remove from mold.
5. Cut the Red soap bar in half and place a piece into each of the two round mold cavities pushing the pieces down and to the side of the mold.
6. Gold soap: You will need ½ cup of melted soap.
7. Add a few drops of fragrance and Gold color powder into melted soap. Stir until well blended.
8. Spray the Red pieces with rubbing alcohol to help the layers adhere to one another.
9. Slowly pour the Gold colored soap along the side of the Red piece. Spray with rubbing alcohol to remove air bubbles.
10. Let soap completely cool. Once soap has completely cooled, release from mold by applying constant, even pressure with thumbs on the back of the mold.
11. Wrap each of the four bars in plastic wrap.
12. Place 2 bars together, alternating the colors. Tie bars together with ribbon.

Citrus Slice Soap

Add a bit of zest to your bath with Citrus Slice soap bars. These lemon and lime scented soaps will perk up your attitude and brighten your day.

MATERIALS:
lbs. Clear Glycerin Soap Brick - *LOTP 52001*
lbs. White Glycerin Soap Brick - *LOTP 52007*
Liquid Soap Colorant - *LOTP*
Soap Fragrance - *LOTP*

SUPPLIES:
Soap Kettle/Ladle - *LOTP 40000*
TIP: A microwave oven can be used instead of the soap kettle.
PVC or a 4-Shape Bar Mold (Use the round cavity of the mold only) - *LOTP 15154*
Wooden craft sticks or spoon
Cutting board
Glass measuring cups
Kitchen knife
Rubbing alcohol in a spray bottle
Plastic wrap
Scissors

SOAP KETTLE INSTRUCTIONS:
1. Cut Clear soap brick into cubes with knife and place into Soap Kettle.
2. Melt soap in Soap Kettle, following manufacturer's instructions.

MICROWAVE INSTRUCTIONS:
1. Cut Clear soap brick into cubes, and place into a microwave-safe measuring cup.
2. Heat for 40 seconds, then in 10-second intervals until soap is completely melted. Stir between melting intervals.

PREPARE CITRUS SLICES:
1. You will need approximately ½ cup of melted Clear soap for each color used.
2. Add a few drops of fragrance and liquid colorant to melted soap. Stir until well blended.
3. Fill the round cavity of the 4-shape bar mold. Spray lightly with rubbing alcohol to dissipate any surface bubbles.
4. Let the soap bar set completely. Release bars from mold by applying constant even pressure with thumbs on the back of mold.
5. Trim the diameter of soap bar approximately ⅛" all the way around the bar.
6. Place the trimmed round bar onto cutting board and slice 4 times; similar to slicing pizza; to get 8 equal slices.
7. Place 8 slices, pointy tip to center, back into the same round cavity of mold. Space evenly to fill circle.
8. Follow melting instructions to melt approximately ⅓ cup of White soap base.
9. Add a few drops of fragrance and liquid colorant to melted soap. Stir until well blended.
10. Do Not overheat the opaque mixture. If soap is bubbling, allow it to cool a bit or it will melt your slices. Pour melted soap to fill the

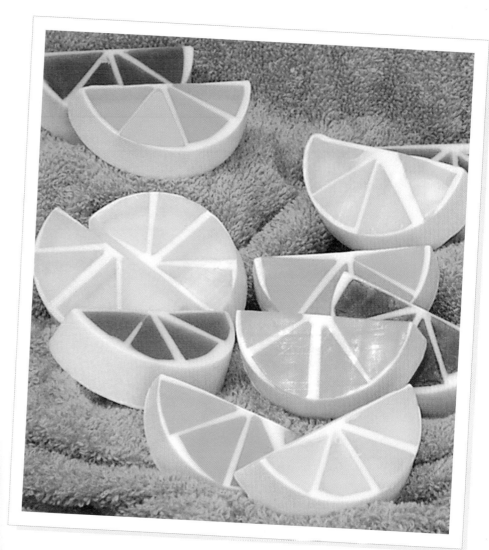

round cavity mold around slices.
11. Let the soap bar set completely. Release bars from mold by applying constant even pressure with thumbs on the back of the mold.
12. Wrap immediately in plastic wrap to preserve freshness until ready to use.

TIPS: • Use Transparent Orange, Yellow and Lime Green soaps for fruit slices.
• Place pipe with hardened soap in freezer to chill to make soap removal easier.
• Remember to let hot white soap cool a bit before pouring it around fruit slices so the colored portion will not melt.
• Make a plunger with a 1½" circle of heavy cardboard and a stick.

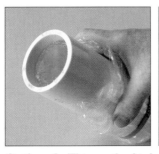 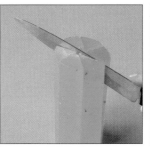 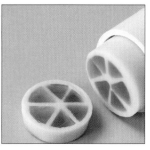

Optional: This method takes more preparation, but is great for making lots of bars.'
1. Sand outside ends of a PVC pipe . Rubber band 8 layers of plastic wrap on one end of 2" pipe. Pour in colored transparent soap, allow to harden • 2. Push soap out end of pipe with a plunger. Cut fruit in half lengthwise. Cut halves in thirds. Do not mix up the sections. Place 8 layers of plastic wrap on work surface. Arrange 6 sections in center of plastic. Keep the soap sections spaced a bit apart. Do not try to be too perfect. Place 3" pipe over sections. Carefully bring plastic wrap up around sides of pipe and secure with the rubber band. • 3. Melt and pour Opaque White. Allow to harden. Place in freezer to cool. Remove the soap from the pipe and slice fruit sections.

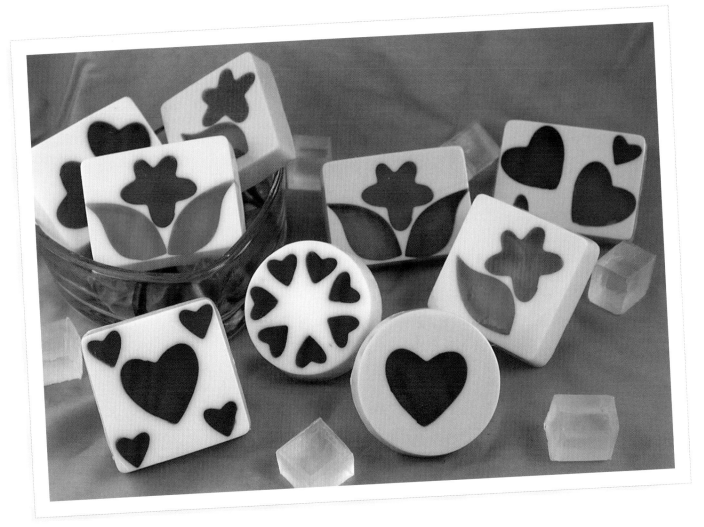

Cookie Cutter Soap

Create a unique line of designer soaps in fun cookie cutter shapes.

MATERIALS:
2 lbs. Clear Glycerin Soap Brick
  - *LOTP 52001*
2 lbs. White Glycerin Soap Brick
  - *LOTP 52007*
Liquid or Powder Colorant - *LOTP*
Soap Fragrance - *LOTP*
Fondant cookie cutters - *Wilton*

SUPPLIES:
Soap Kettle/Ladle - *LOTP 40000*
TIP: A microwave oven can be used
  instead of the soap kettle.
4-Shape Bar Mold - *LOTP 15154*
Wooden craft sticks
  or spoon for stirring
Cutting board
Microwave safe glass measuring cups
Kitchen knife
Rubbing alcohol in a spray bottle
Plastic wrap
Scissors
Optional decorative paper
Optional ribbon or raffia

SOAP KETTLE MELTING INSTRUCTIONS:
1. Cut Clear soap brick into cubes.
2. Melt soap in Soap Kettle following manufacturer's instructions.

MICROWAVE MELTING INSTRUCTIONS:
1. Cut Clear soap brick into cubes. Place into a measuring cup.
2. Heat for 40 seconds, then in 10-second intervals until soap is completely melted, stirring between intervals.

PREPARING SOAP CUTOUT PIECES:
1. You will need ¼ cup per bar of melted Clear soap for each color used. Place melted soap in measuring cup.
2. Add a few drops of fragrance and your first colorant in small amounts. Stir until blended.
3. Pick a cavity in the 4-shape bar mold into which the cutout will fit. Slowly pour melted soap until cavity is about half full. Spray lightly with rubbing alcohol.
4. If you are using another color for cutouts, repeat the above steps to fill other cavities with different colors.
5. Let set completely, about 30 minutes.
6. Release bars from mold by applying constant pressure with thumbs on the back of mold.
7. Using the Cookie or Fondant cutters, press the cutter through the bar and remove soap from the center of the cutter.

PREPARING BACKGROUND OPAQUE BAR:
1. Melt White soap following the melting instructions. You will need slightly less than ¼ cup of melted White soap for each soap bar.
2. Place soap cutout pieces into mold cavities creating a design. Press firmly to mold so that when you pour White soap on top of it, it will not seep under pieces.
3. Add a few drops of fragrance and colorant to melted White soap. Stir until well blended.
4. Make sure the White soap is not overheated or it will melt your pieces. Pour melted soap into the mold over the cutout pieces, filling the cavity completely.
5. Cool completely. Release from mold by applying constant even pressure with thumbs on the back of the mold.
6. Tightly wrap soap bars in plastic wrap.

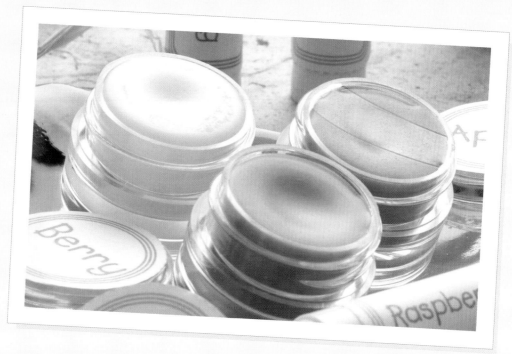

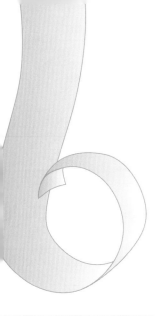
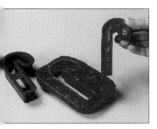
Lip Balms and Glosses

Make deliciously fruity lip balms, and shiny lip-gloss canisters that will look so good no one will believe you made them yourself!

MATERIALS:
Lip Balm Mixture - *LOTP*
Lip Gloss Mixture - *LOTP*
Lip Flavoring - *LOTP*
Color Powder - *LOTP*

SUPPLIES:
Lip Canisters - *LOTP*
Microwave oven
Wooden craft sticks or spoons
2-cup glass measuring cup or glass bowl
Disposable medicine dropper or pipette

Optional: decorative labels

Lip Gloss

LIP GLOSS INSTRUCTIONS:
1. To make more than one color, split contents of gloss in half and continue. Using the plastic tub that the lip balm already comes in as your mixing bowl, add powder colorant in pinches until desired shade has been reached. Mix after each addition.
2. Add flavoring a few drops at a time, mixing after each addition, until desired effect has been reached.

Lip Balm

LIP BALM INSTRUCTIONS:
1. Empty contents of the sunflower oil and beeswax beads into a microwave-safe measuring cup.
2. Microwave in 30 second intervals until beads are completely melted. Stir contents between melting intervals.
3. At this point, if you are making 2 colors, divide the mixture into 2 separate measuring cups.
4. Add flavoring a drop at a time and stir until desired effect has been achieved.
5. Add color powder in small amounts and stir until you attain the desired color.
6. Using plastic pipette or dropper, transfer lip balm to the tubes or canisters. Fill each container to the rim. (If pipette gets clogged with dried lip balm, simply run 2 fingers down the side of the pipette while pushing the excess lip balm out of the opened end.)
7. Allow the mixture to settle for a few minutes, and then add another drop. This drop prevents holes that will occasionally form in the center of the tube.
8. Allow the mixture to set for 20-30 minutes before you move it or put the lids on.
9. Adhere a decorative label.

Design Tips:

Layers: Pour mixture about ⅓ full and let harden. Pour second color another ⅓ and let harden. Using first color, fill canister or tube to the top.

Bulls-eye Design: Pour mixture into a canister, about ⅓ full. Let mixture harden for a few minutes, then place the cap on the tube in the center of the canister, open side up. Fill the canister the rest of the way and let harden.

Once lip balm is hard, remove the lid from the center and fill the opening with second color. Let harden 20 minutes, and put lid on top.

If mixture sets between pours in your measuring cup, microwave for 30 seconds to liquefy it.

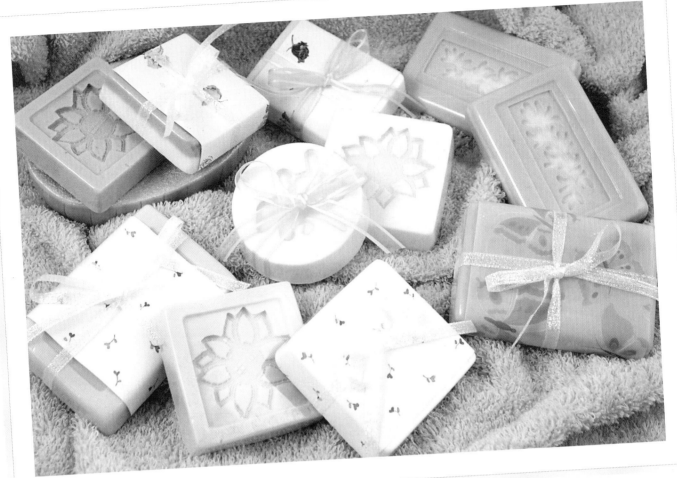

Embossed Soap Bars

The Embossed Soap Kit includes everything needed to complete the project. The mold is reusable and the border on the bars gives the finished soaps a professional designer look.

MATERIALS:
Embossed Soap Kit - *LOTP 57020*
- OR -
    2 lbs. Clear Glycerin Soap Brick - *LOTP 52001*
    4-Shape Bar Mold - *LOTP 15154*
    2 lbs. White Glycerin Soap Brick - *LOTP 52007*
    Liquid Soap Colorant or Powder Soap Colorant - *LOTP*
    Soap Fragrance - *LOTP*
    Rubber Stamps

SUPPLIES:
Soap Kettle/Ladle - *LOTP 40000*
    TIP: A microwave can be used instead of the soap kettle.
Wooden craft sticks or spoon for stirring
Cutting board
Glass measuring cups
Kitchen knife
Rubbing alcohol in a spray bottle
Plastic wrap
Scissors
Optional decorative paper
Optional ribbon or raffia

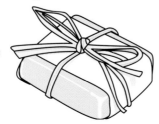

SOAP KETTLE MELTING
INSTRUCTIONS:
1. Cut Clear soap brick into cubes.
2. Melt soap in Soap Kettle following manufacturer's instructions.

MICROWAVE MELTING
INSTRUCTIONS:
1. Cut Clear soap brick into cubes, and place into a microwave-safe measuring cup.
2. Heat for 40 seconds, then in 10-second intervals until soap is completely melted. Stir between melting intervals.

INSTRUCTIONS:
1. You will need approximately ½ cup of melted Clear or White soap for each soap bar.
2. Add a few drops of fragrance to melted soap and stir until well blended.
3. Add a few drops of liquid colorant or add small amounts of powder colorant to melted White soap and stir until well blended and desired color has been reached.
4. Pour a small drop of soap into the mold and affix the stamp, design facing up, into the mold. This will hold stamp in place when soap is poured into the mold. Press firmly so stamp adheres to surface.
5. Fill the mold with melted, colored, fragrant soap mixture.
6. Let harden and remove from mold. To remove stamp from soap bar simply lift a corner slowly and pull back until stamp is completely removed from soap.
7. Wrap soap in decorative paper and tie with ribbon or raffia.

Helpful Recipes for Herbal Bars

Herbal bars contain ingredients that cleanse, condition and heal the skin. Just choose herbs that match your skin type.

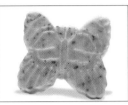

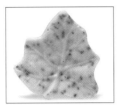

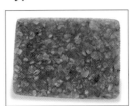

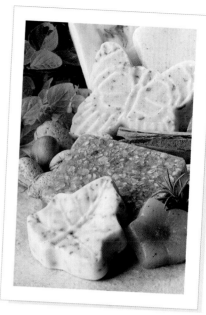

Almond Soap

Almond soap is a good cleanser and can unclog pores in the face.

Grind ½ cup of almonds into chunks, remove half and grind remaining nuts into a meal. Add almonds, fragrance and an extra tablespoon of oil to the Basic Hand Milled Soap Recipe. Mold. Almond oil may be substituted for olive oil.

Mint Soap

This soap has a fresh, stimulating smell.

Brew ¼ cup of water with mint leaves. Discard leaves from mint water. Add mint water, ¼ cup of dried mint and 1 to 2 drops of Green colorant to the Basic Hand Milled Soap Recipe. Add dried mint leaves for color.

Oatmeal Soap

This soap can gently soften sensitive skin.

Gently fold ¼ cup of oatmeal and cinnamon scent drops into melted soap. Or hand mill the soap.

Milk & Honey Soap

Honey is a natural emollient, milk is a cleanser. This age-old combination promotes healthy skin.

Add 2 tablespoons of powdered milk, 2 tablespoons of honey, 3 tablespoons of water and a dash of nutmeg for color to the Basic Hand Milled Soap Recipe. A little citronella enhances the honey fragrance of this soft soap.

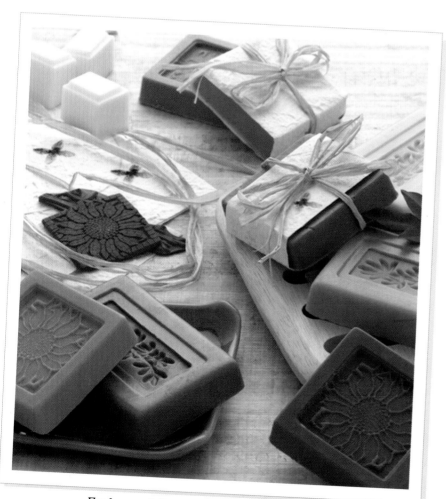

Embossed Soap Bars in Earth Colors

Basic Hand Milled Soap Recipe

MATERIALS:
2 lbs. Clear Glycerin Soap Brick - *LOTP 52007*
2 tablespoons water
2 tablespoons olive oil
Liquid Soap Colorant - *LOTP*
Soap Fragrance - *LOTP*

Prepare ingredients in three containers:
1. soap cubes, 2. liquids (water, oil & fragrance), 3. dry ingredients.• Melt cubes of soap in microwave. Allow soap to stop steaming before removing. • Add oil, water, botanicals, fragrance and colors to a bowl. • Whisk vigorously until soap thickens to the consistency of heavy cream. • Beat until mixture is fluffy (it will look like egg whites). Pour mixture into mold, let harden. • Remove shapes from mold, place on a rack to dry. Air dry for 2 weeks.

- Hand milled soaps have a natural, hand made look.
- The soaps last longer and are usually more expensive than other soaps.
- If soap becomes too sudsy while beating, add more oil.
- It requires more colorant for hand milled soap.

Additives and Fragrances

- Use any fragrance that is added to candles, soap or potpourri.
- Do not use perfumes that are alcohol based. The fragrance will evaporate.
- Fruit Fresh can be added to soaps with fresh fruits and vegetables as a preservative.

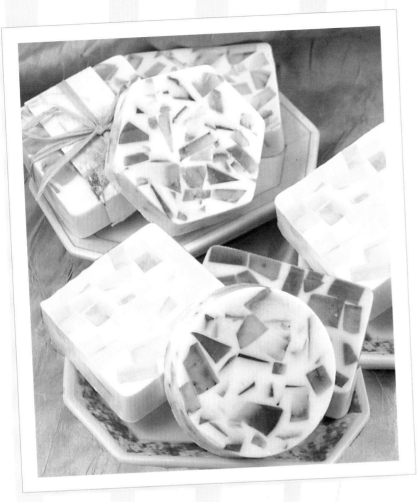

Soap Chunk Bars

Create fun Soap Chunk Bars by suspending colorful bits of soap inside. This is a great project to use up all your colorful left-over scraps from other projects.

Helpful Hints

Place small soap pieces in the freezer to chill to prevent melting when hot soap is added. • Make as many layers as desired to spread the chunks and pieces throughout the soap. • Use slightly cooled liquid soap as the base to keep from melting the chunks and pieces.

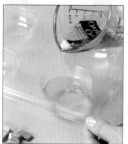 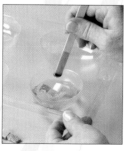 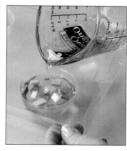

1. Cut small chunks of colored soap and place in a freezer to chill. Melt base soap. • 2. Pour half of base soap into mold and add a portion of the small chunks. Allow a skin to form on top. • 3. Place the second half of small chunks on the skimmed surface. Slowly pour on slightly cooled base soap.

MATERIALS:
2 lbs. Clear Glycerin Soap Brick - *LOTP 52001*
2 lbs. White Glycerin Soap Brick - *LOTP 52007*
Liquid Soap Colorant - *LOTP*
Soap Fragrance - *LOTP*

SUPPLIES:
Soap Kettle/Ladle - *LOTP 40000*
 TIP: A microwave oven can be used
 instead of the soap kettle.
4-Shape Bar Mold - *LOTP 15154*
Wooden craft sticks or spoon
Cutting board
Glass measuring cups
Rubbing alcohol in a spray bottle
Plastic wrap • Kitchen knife • Scissors
Optional: decorative paper, ribbon or raffia.

SOAP KETTLE MELTING INSTRUCTIONS:
1. Cut Clear soap brick into cubes.
2. Melt soap in Soap Kettle following manufacturer's instructions.

MICROWAVE MELTING INSTRUCTIONS:
1. Cut Clear soap brick into cubes, and place into a microwave-safe measuring cup.
2. Heat for 40 seconds, then in 10-second intervals until soap is completely melted. Stir between melting intervals.

PREPARE CHUNK SOAP:
1. You will need ½ cup of melted Clear soap for each color used.
2. Add a few drops of fragrance and liquid colorant to melted soap. Stir until well blended.
3. Pour into the 4-shape bar mold filling one of the cavities completely. Spray lightly with rubbing alcohol.
4. If you'd like to fill all 4 mold cavities with different colors, follow above instructions using a different color for each cavity.
5. Let set completely.
6. Proceed to Step 1 of Soap Chunk Bars.
7. Release bars from mold by applying constant even pressure with thumbs on the back of the mold.
8. Cut each soap bar into small chunks with knife.
9. Proceed to Step 3 of Soap Chunk Bars.

SOAP CHUNK BARS:
1. Melt White soap following the melting instructions. You will need approximately ½ cup of melted White soap for each soap bar.
2. Go to Step 7 of Prepare Chunk Soap.
3. Add a few drops of fragrance and liquid colorant to melted White soap. Stir until well blended.
4. Pour a small amount of melted soap into one cavity of the 4-shape bar mold, just enough to cover the bottom, and spray with rubbing alcohol.
5. Spray soap chunks with rubbing alcohol and carefully scatter a layer of soap chunks into the mold cavity, over melted soap. To prevent air pockets and allow melted soap to flow around and under chunks, spray mold cavity with rubbing alcohol, Be sure to spray all chunk surfaces.
6. Pour enough melted soap to almost cover chunks and spray again with rubbing alcohol.
7. Repeat steps 5-6 until mold is filled. Let cool completely.
8. Release from mold by applying constant even pressure with thumbs on the back of the mold.
9. Tightly wrap soap bars in plastic wrap.
10. Wrap decorative paper around finished soap bar and tie a pretty ribbon or raffia around the bar.

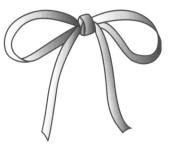

Rock Soap Bars

SOAP KETTLE
MELTING INSTRUCTIONS:
1. Cut Clear soap brick into cubes.
2. Melt soap in Soap Kettle following manufacturer's instructions.

MICROWAVE
MELTING INSTRUCTIONS:
1. Cut Clear soap brick into cubes, and place into a microwave-safe measuring cup.
2. Heat for 40 seconds, then in 10-second intervals until soap is completely melted. Stir between melting intervals.

INSTRUCTIONS:
1. You will need ½ cup of melted Clear soap for each color used in a 3-color soap rock.
2. Add a few drops of fragrance to melted soap, and stir until well blended.
3. Add liquid or powder colorant in small amounts until desired color is reached. For a more dramatic look, use both liquid and powder colorant together.
4. Alternating between all colors being used, pour thin uneven layers of soap.
　　Prop the mold up slightly and rotate when changing colors. This will ensure a more uneven, natural look.
　　Let layers briefly harden before pouring more color so colors don't totally blend together.
　　If soap hardens too much before pouring the next layer, spray soap with alcohol so the layers adhere to one another. Fill the mold.
5. Let cool completely. Release by applying constant even pressure with thumbs on the back of the mold.
　　Carve into desired rock shapes.

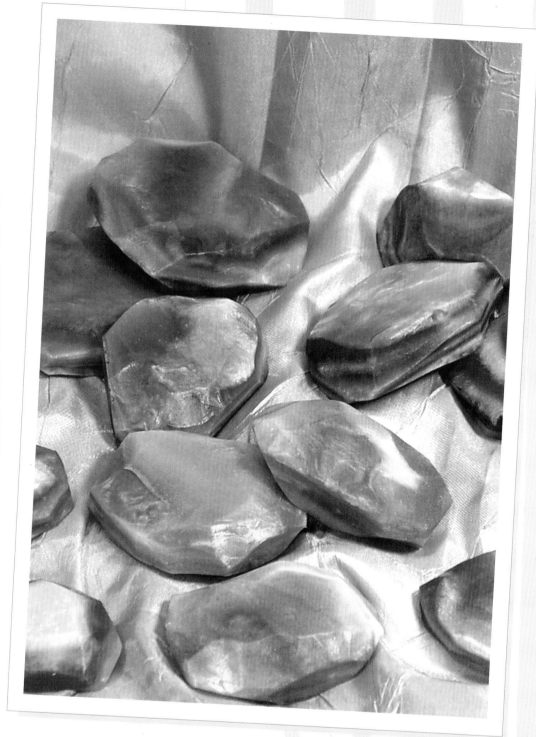

Rock Soap Bars

Carved Rock Soap Bars are each as unique as their natural look-alikes. No two will ever be the same.

Save the left-over soap bits to make Chunk Soap Bars on page 12.

MATERIALS:
2 lbs. Clear Glycerin Soap Brick - *LOTP 52001*
　Optional 2 lbs. White Glycerin Soap Brick - *LOTP 52007*
Liquid or Powder Soap Colorant - *LOTP*
Soap Fragrance - *LOTP*

SUPPLIES:
Soap Kettle/Ladle - *LOTP 40000*
　TIP: A microwave oven can be used instead of the soap kettle.
4-Shape Bar Mold - *LOTP 15154*
Wooden craft sticks or spoon for stirring
Cutting board
Glass measuring cups
Kitchen knife
Rubbing alcohol in a spray bottle
Plastic wrap
Scissors

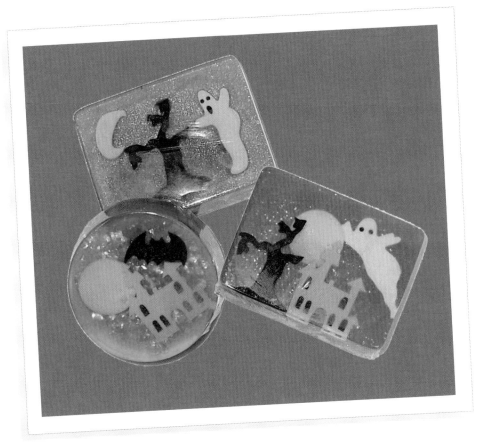

There is no need to discard any scraps you cut from the soap rolls or bars.

Simply cut them into chunks and use the pieces to make Chunk Bar Soaps on page 12.

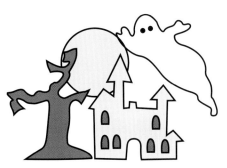

Spooky Halloween Foam Soap Bars

Scare up some excitement and fun with Spooky Halloween Foam Soap Bars.

MATERIALS:
2 lbs. Clear Glycerin Soap Brick
   - *LOTP 52001*
Liquid Soap Colorants - *LOTP*
Soap Fragrance - *LOTP*
Soap Glitter - *LOTP*

SUPPLIES:
Soap Kettle/Ladle - *LOTP 40000*
4-Shape Bar Mold - *LOTP 15154*
Halloween Shapes made of Craft Foam
Wooden craft sticks or spoons
Glass measuring cup
Kitchen knife
Rubbing alcohol in a spray bottle
Toothpicks
Plastic wrap
Scissors

PREPARATION:
Arrange halloween foam pieces into scenes that will fit into the mold cavities. Arrange a scene for each mold cavity before preparing soap.

SOAP KETTLE MELTING INSTRUCTIONS:
1. Cut Clear soap brick into cubes.
2. Melt soap in Soap Kettle following manufacturer's instructions.

MICROWAVE MELTING INSTRUCTIONS:
1. Cut Clear soap brick into cubes and place into a microwave-safe measuring cup.
2. Heat for 40 seconds, then in 10-second intervals until soap is completely melted. Stir between melting intervals.

HALLOWEEN SOAP BARS;
1. Ladle approximately ½ cup of melted soap into glass measuring cup.
2. Add fragrance to melted soap and stir until well incorporated. Do Not add color.
3. Working rather quickly, pour melted soap into one of the mold cavities, until it is ⅓ full.
4. Immediately spray foam pieces, front and back with rubbing alcohol and place face down into the mold cavity, on top of the poured soap.
   Tap the foam pieces gently and spray again with rubbing alcohol. The rubbing alcohol is used to prevent air pockets. Use toothpicks to gently hold the foam pieces in place if they move around.
5. Repeat steps 5-6 for all mold cavities.
6. Let soap set, almost completely, for approximately 5 minutes.
7. Ladle approximately 1 cup of melted Clear soap into glass measuring cup.
8. Add liquid colorant, fragrance and glitter to melted soap. Stir until well blended.
9. Spray all four mold cavities with rubbing alcohol and pour melted soap into each cavity until full.
10. Spray all with rubbing alcohol.
11. Let soap set completely.
12. Release by applying constant even pressure with your thumbs on the back of the mold.
13. Tightly wrap soap bars in plastic wrap.

Fishy Foam Soap Bars

PREPARATION:
Arrange fish foam pieces into scenes that will fit into the mold cavities. Arrange a scene for each mold cavity before preparing soap.

SOAP KETTLE
MELTING INSTRUCTIONS:
1. Cut Clear soap brick into cubes.
2. Melt soap in Soap Kettle following manufacturer's instructions.

MICROWAVE
MELTING INSTRUCTIONS:
1. Cut Clear soap brick into cubes and place into a microwave-safe measuring cup.
2. Heat for 40 seconds, then in 10-second intervals until soap is completely melted. Stir between melting intervals.

FISH SOAP BARS:
1. Stir fragrance into melted soap as desired.
2. Pour a small amount of the Clear melted soap into one of the mold cavities, pouring only enough to fill approximately 1/4 of the mold. Spray poured soap with rubbing alcohol to remove air bubbles.
3. Immediately spray the first foam fish scene with rubbing alcohol and place it face down into the poured, melted soap. Spray again with rubbing alcohol.
4. Continue, repeating steps 2-3 until all mold cavities are filled. If foam pieces move out of place, use a toothpick to gently center them.
5. Let the soap and foam scenes set for approximately 5 minutes until a thin layer of skin has formed.
6. Spray with rubbing alcohol and pour a thin layer of Clear melted soap over the foam pieces. Pour just enough to cover them completely and let set for approximately 3-5 minutes. If Clear soap has set up in the measuring cup, re-melt it in the microwave.
7. Prepare the colored soap for the back of the bar. Melt Clear or White soap following melting instructions.
8. Stir fragrance and liquid soap colorant into the melted soap, a couple drops at a time, until desired effect has been achieved.
9. Spray mold cavities with rubbing alcohol and pour colored soap into each of the cavities until they are all filled. Spray with rubbing alcohol.
10. Allow soap to cool completely. Remove bars by applying constant pressure on the back of the mold.
11. Wrap soap bars in Clear plastic wrap to preserve their freshness.

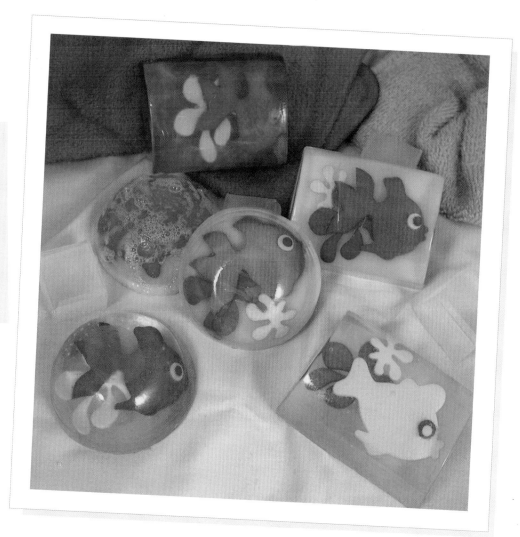

Fishy Foam Soap Bars

Fishy Foam Soaps are imaginative decorations for the kid's bath or as fun favors for a child's birthday party.

MATERIALS:
2 lbs. Clear Glycerin Soap Brick - *LOTP 52001*
2 lbs. White Glycerin Soap Brick - *LOTP 52007*
Soap Dyes - *LOTP 53001*
Cucumber Melon Fragrance - *LOTP 51026*

SUPPLIES:
Darice Foam Fish Shapes
Soap Kettle/Ladle - *LOTP 40000*
    TIP: A microwave oven can be used instead of the soap kettle.
Oval Round Mold - *LOTP 15152*
    OR Dome Bar Mold - *LOTP 15168*
Microwave-safe measuring cup
Kitchen knife
Spoon or craft stick for mixing
Rubbing alcohol in a spray bottle
Cutting board
Plastic wrap
Scissors
Toothpicks

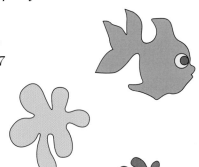
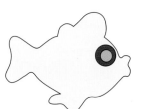

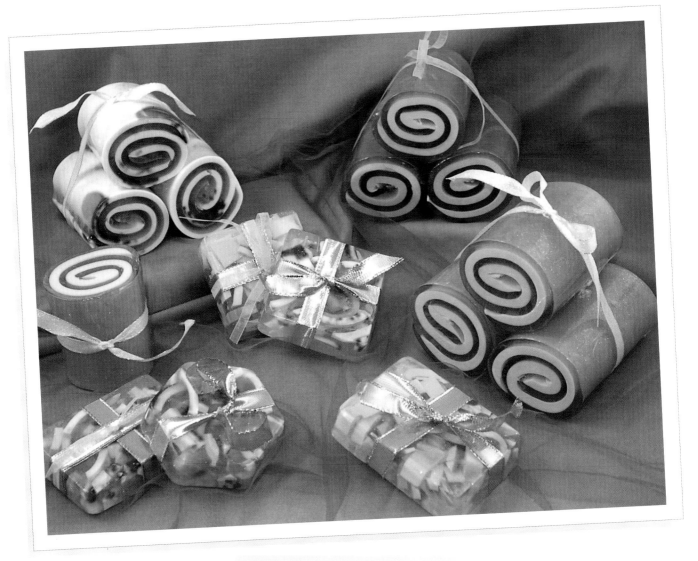

Soap Rolls

Sweet smelling and delightful, these soap rolls turn a soap dish into something special.

MATERIALS:
Liquid Soap Colorants - *LOTP*
Soap Fragrance - *LOTP*
2 lbs. Clear Glycerin Soap Brick - *LOTP 52001*
2 lbs. White Glycerin Soap Brick - *LOTP 52007*

SUPPLIES:
Raffia or paper ribbon
Soap Kettle/Ladle - *LOTP 40000*
4-Shape Bar Mold - *LOTP 15154*
Wilton 10½" x 15½" cookie/jelly roll baking sheet pan
Wooden craft sticks or spoons
2-cup glass measuring cup or glass bowl
Kitchen knife
Rubbing alcohol in a spray bottle
Plastic wrap • Scissors

SOAP KETTLE MELTING INSTRUCTIONS:
1. Cut Clear soap brick into cubes.
2. Melt soap in Soap Kettle following manufacturer's instructions.

MICROWAVE MELTING INSTRUCTIONS:
1. Cut Clear soap brick into cubes and place into a microwave-measuring cup.
2. Heat for 40 seconds, then in 10-second intervals until soap is completely melted. Stir between melting intervals.

INSTRUCTIONS:
1. Carefully ladle approximately 2 cups of melted soap into a large glass measuring cup or glass bowl.
2. Add fragrance to melted soap and stir until well blended. Add a small amount of color if desired.
3. Pour melted soap onto cookie sheet and spray with rubbing alcohol to remove air bubbles.
4. Let soap set, almost completely, for approximately 15 minutes.
5. While you are waiting for soap to set, repeat steps 1 through 3 using the White soap brick.
6. Add liquid colorant and fragrance to

White melted soap, stir until well blended.
7. Spray the soap that has set in the cookie sheet with rubbing alcohol to adhere layer.
8. Immediately pour melted soap onto the cookie sheet over the Clear soap. When pouring this layer, pour soap all around the sheet. Do Not pour in one spot, or the soap in that area may melt. Spray with alcohol again.
9. Let soap set, approximately 15 minutes. Not let soap set completely. It must be slightly warm and pliable in order to roll the soap.
10. Cut soap away from the sides with knife and remove from cookie sheet.
11. Cut soap into short strips, cutting from long side of soap up.
12. Working quickly, take one strip and place on a clean surface with the Clear side down. Cut edge closest to you at a 45-degree angle.
13. Bend the cut edge over once and press down a bit. Roll soap as tightly as possible.
14. When you get close to the end of roll, cut the edge at a 45-degree angle, finish rolling.
15. Repeat steps 14 through 16 using the remaining soap strips.
16. Cut soap rolls with a knife on each side, make neat slice.
17. Tightly wrap soap rolls in plastic wrap.
18. Tie pretty paper ribbon or raffia around individual rolls or stacks of rolls.

Bath Bomb Balls

INSTRUCTIONS:

Please be sure to read all directions completely before beginning this project.

. **Prepare mold:** Cut each cavity from the mold leaving a small ½" edge around each dome.

. Pour the contents of both powder Bath Bomb Mixes into a bowl or measuring cup and mix well. Separate the mixture into 2 equal parts and set aside.

Once powder ingredients are mixed together, they are extremely sensitive to moisture. If you do not plan on making both bombs at once, store in an airtight container in a cool, dry place.

. **Choose** the color and fragrance. See Coloring Tips for mixing colors.

Pour approximately ¼ of the bottle of liquid colorant, ¼ of the bottle of fragrance and ¼ ounce of water into the spray bottle. Using less water in your spray bottle will concentrate the color.

. **Spray** 3 squirts of the liquid into the pre-measured powder mix. Mix well. Continue until the mix is wet enough to pack it together. Don't wet the mix too much or it will expand; if it does, just add a little more dry powder to the mix.

. **Fill** 2 mold cavities with the moistened powder mixture, packing tightly and overfilling them lightly.

. **Press** both halves together and squeeze them tightly. Promptly begin to gently remove one of the plastic molds from the bath bomb.

Turn the bomb over into your hand and gently remove the second plastic mold.

Smooth out the seam by softly rubbing with the back side of a spoon. Handle gently as the mix is not yet hardened. Place on a smooth surface to dry.

. **Rinse** out the spray bottle. Repeat steps 3-6 above for another bath bomb.

. Allow bath bombs to completely harden - about 24 hours. Place bath bomb in a clear bag and personalize with decorative labels and ribbon.

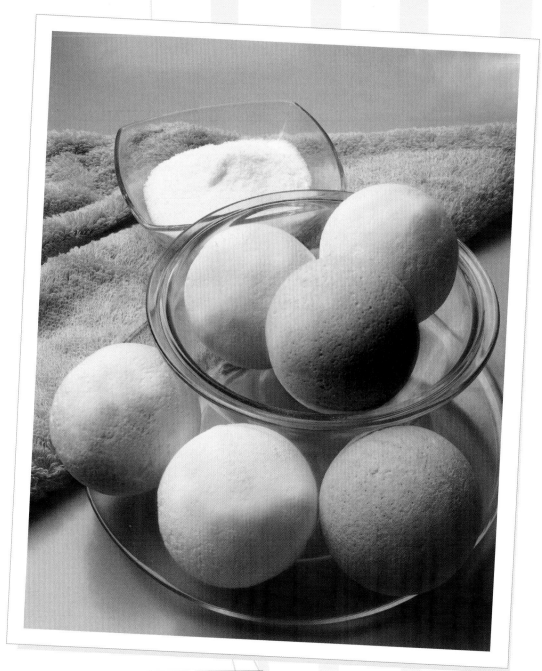

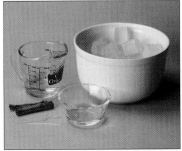
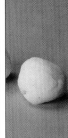

Coloring Tips:

Red + Yellow = Orange

Blue + Red = Purple

Blue + Yellow = Green

Or create your own colors—mix a few drops in a small cup of water first to test.

Bath Bomb Balls

Bring the spa experience into your home with these great bath bombs. Your friends will love these as gifts.

MATERIALS:
Liquid Soap Colorant - *LOTP*
Soap Fragrance - *LOTP*
Fizzie Mix Refill pack - *LOTP*
(Bath Bomb Mixes)

SUPPLIES:
Round ball mold - *LOTP M68*
Spray bottle
Wooden craft sticks or spoon
Glass measuring cups

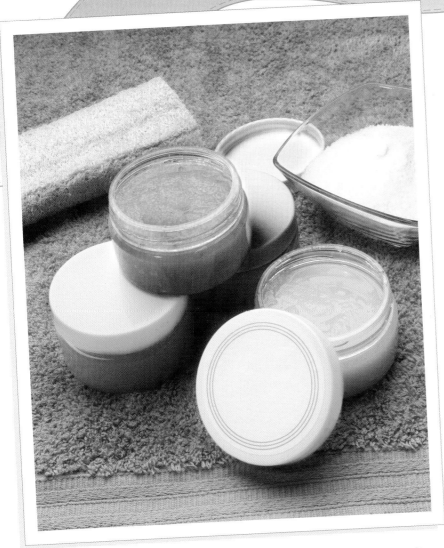

Sugar Scrub

Sugar Cane produces glycolic acid, one of the natural alpha hydroxy acids that exfoliates the skin. Sugar scrubs leave your skin feeling so incredibly soft, you will want to use it all over.

MATERIALS:
Liquid Soap Colorant - *LOTP*
Soap Fragrance - *LOTP*
White granulated sugar
Sunflower oil
    OR Sugar & Salt Scrub Kit - *LOTP*

SUPPLIES:
Jars for storing finished scrubs (included in kit)
Spoon for stirring
Glass measuring cup or mixing bowl

INSTRUCTIONS:
1. Pour 1 lb. of granulated sugar into a mixing bowl or measuring cup.
2. Slowly add 6 ounces of sunflower oil into the sugar, stirring continuously.
3. Add 3-4 drops of fragrance into the scrub mixture. Stir the fragrance through and continue adding fragrance a few drops at a time until desired fragrance has been reached.
4. Add 3-4 drops of color into the mixture, stirring continuously. Continue adding color and mixing until desired color has been reached.
5. Spoon mixture into the containers.
6. Adhere a decorative label.

Bath Salts in a Bottle

Fabulous and Soothing…Salts and oils add enjoyment and aid relaxation as you bathe.

MATERIALS:
1 cup of Epsom salt
1 cup of sea or rock salt
    or 32 oz. Bath Salts
    - *LOTP 61007*
Food coloring
    or Liquid Soap Colorant - *LOTP*
20 drops of Soap Fragrance - *LOTP*

INSTRUCTIONS:
1. Empty salts into an airtight glass jar.
2. Add fragrance, a couple drops at a time, mixing after each addition.
3. Add liquid colorant, a few drops at a time, mixing after each addition.
4. Use 1/4 cup per bath for a relaxing aromatic experience.

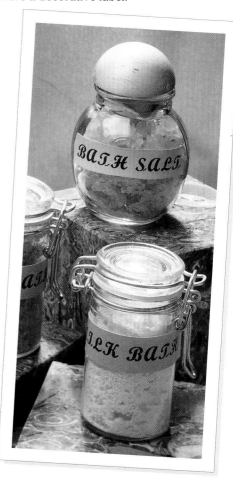

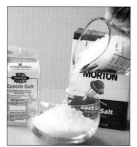 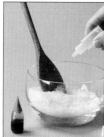 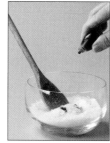 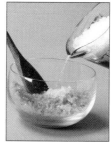

1. Measure Epsom and rock salt, pour into a bowl. • 2. Add fragrance and stir. • 3. Add color and mix until all salt is colored. • 4. Add additional salt if mixture is too damp.